# *HomeBirth Education*

## Deborah Duren-Smithey, CPM

Information in this book shall not take the place of
the advice of your healthcare provider.

# Contents

# Congratulations!

Now is an exciting time to be expecting a baby. There is a reason your baby is coming at this moment in history. Your job is to do the best you can to grow the strongest, healthiest baby possible to give him or her the best start you can.

# Why Homebirth?

Every woman has the inalienable right to choose where, how and with whom she will birth her baby. Birth is not an isolated event in a woman's life. It is a spiritual, psycho/social, physical passage which affects not only the rest of her life and her self-concept but the lives of her family and community. If you are expecting a child, you carry the future within you! You deserve to be respected and well cared for. There is not one right maternity caregiver for all women but there is a right caregiver for each woman. Each woman must choose what type of caregiver she wants and then shop around and interview a few of that type to find the one that is right for her.

Women birth best where they feel safest. Some feel safest in the hospital, others feel safest at home. It is reassuring that all the valid scientific studies comparing outcomes of midwife-attended homebirth with low-risk hospital birth show the risks are about the same. The satisfaction rate, however, is much higher with homebirth.

# Basic Maternal Anatomy

The mother's womb, or uterus, is the organ in which the baby grows. The opening, at the bottom of the uterus, is called the cervix. The cervix is closed during pregnancy, and must fully open to allow the baby out of the uterus and through the birth canal, or vagina.

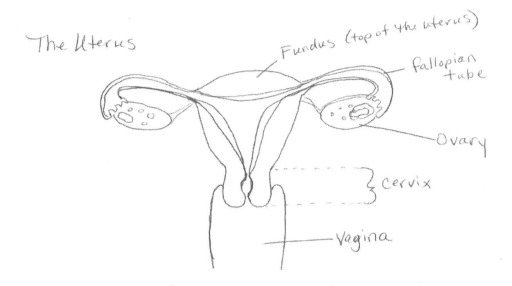

When we talk about birth, it is helpful if we understand the parts of the mother's anatomy that affect birth.

The mother's bony pelvis forms both a cradle that supports the baby during pregnancy and a funnel through which the baby must pass during birth.

In late pregnancy, the hormone "relaxin" causes all the joints and ligaments in the body to loosen and relax. The joints of the pelvis become more mobile and can stretch and enlarge the pelvis as the baby passes through!

Definition: Pelvimetry—measurement of the adequacy of the female pelvis.

The very definition of pelvimetry is condescending and

8

judgmental! Many women are told during a pap-smear or pelvic exam that their pelvis is "inadequate" or that it is too small to have a baby. This is very frightening! But let's think about it a little. Was the assessment done in late pregnancy when the hormone relaxin has released the joints and ligaments so they are at their loosest? What position is the woman in when the assessment is made? Flat on her back or in a full squat? Is the woman bearing down and pressing a large round baby-head through the pelvis when the assessment is made? How can any pelvimetry be accurate? It simply cannot.

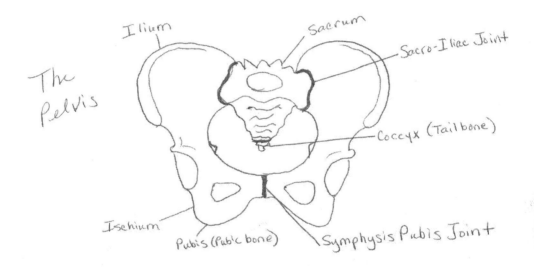

A woman's body knows how to grow a baby. It will not grow a baby too big to birth. Some exceptions that may make it harder or impossible to push the baby through include: junk food diet that grows an unnaturally large baby, history of rickets or scurvy in childhood that deformed the pelvis, car wreck or other trauma that broke the pelvis and it didn't heal right, or out-of-control diabetes.

The skin and muscle between the vaginal opening and the anus is called the perineum. The baby's head stretches the vagina and perineum as it emerges into the world.

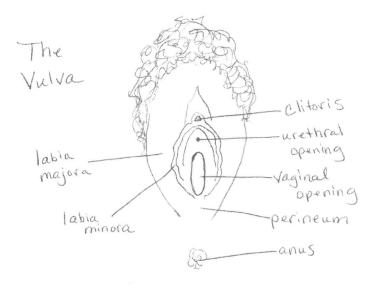

## Baby Skull Anatomy

The bones of the baby's skull shift and mould as the head passes through the mother's bony pelvis. The bones "overlap" and the head re-shapes as it moves through. During infancy and early childhood, the divisions between the bones harden to form a solid skull.

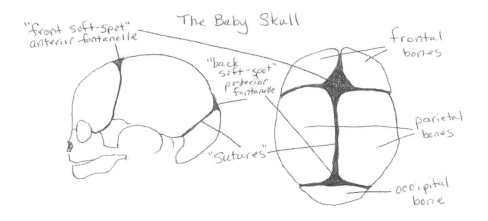

## Emotional Changes

Pregnancy is also a time of emotional change. Not only do the hormones of pregnancy cause mood swings, but fear or apprehension about her ability to cope with the challenge of a new baby may make the mother extra sensitive. All emotions may be amplified during pregnancy.

Avoiding hypoglycemia (low blood sugar) by eating frequent snacks will help to ease some of these mood swings.

Soul-work during early to mid-pregnancy can be very productive. Women can heal many past emotional hang-ups, especially mother-related issues, very effectively during pregnancy. But this work should be put away in the last trimester, when positive affirmations in anticipation of the birth should become the focus.

## Decision-making

As parents, you will make informed decisions for yourself and your baby throughout pregnancy, birth and beyond. Informed decision-making requires research and discussion regarding available testing and treatment for various conditions/occurrences and the risks and benefits of testing/treatment choices. Please ask questions of your midwife, doctor, pastor, and/or other care provider and do your own research so you can feel sure of your decision.

Do the risks of the test, procedure or treatment outweigh the benefits? Only you can make the decision for yourself, your baby and your family, although some practitioners will try to impose their will on you. Governments even "require" some testing, procedures and treatments. Some practitioners will use fear to coerce you into doing what they think is right. Remember, you have a right to decline anything you do not want.

Before consenting to any test, ask yourself:
- What is the benefit of having the results of this test?
- What you would do if the test came back positive? If

it came back negative?
- What would your care provider recommend if the test was positive? Negative?
- Would you continue with the recommendations or decline?
- How would you feel about your choice of action or inaction if there was a poor outcome that was related to your decision?

## *Baby's Lie*

The baby's "lie" is the relationship of the baby's body to the mother's body. The lie can be:
- Longitudinal: when the length of the baby's body is parallel to the length of the mother's body. 99.5% of babies are in a longitudinal lie.
- Transverse: when the length of the baby's body is perpendicular to the length of your body. The baby is "sideways" inside your uterus.
- Oblique: when the length of the baby's body is at an angle to the length of your body, the baby is not straight in line, nor is it perpendicular. It's lying at an angle.

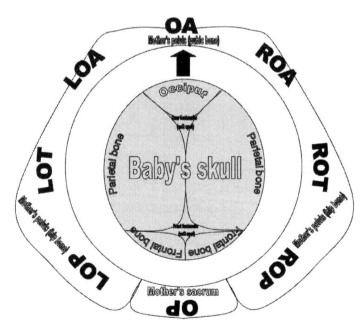

# Baby's Position

The baby's position is determined by the position of the back of the baby in relation to the mother. The reference point in head-down presentation (the most common presentation) is the baby's Occipital Bone (back of the baby's skull).

- OA—occiput anterior, baby's back in line with the front of the mother
- ROA—right occiput anterior, baby's back in line with right-front of mother
- ROT-right occiput transverse, baby's back in line with the mother's right
- ROP—right occiput posterior, baby's back in line with right-rear of mother
- OP—occiput posterior, baby's back straight in in line with mother's back. Birth in this position causes painful "back labor."
- LOP—left occiput posterior, baby's back in line with left-rear of mother
- LOT—left occiput transverse, baby's back in line with mother's right
- LOA—left occiput anterior, baby's back in line with left-front of mother

# Baby's Presentation

The baby's presentation is determined by which part of the baby is descending into the mother's pelvis. It can be:

- Cephalic—the baby's head is coming first. This is the most common presentation. Cephalic presentations can be:
  - Vertex—the baby's head is flexed, the top/back of the baby's head comes out first
  - Sincipital—the baby's head is not very well flexed, the top of the baby's head comes out first
  - Brow—the baby's head is not flexed at all, the baby's brow leads the way
  - Face—the baby's head is tilted strongly toward the back, and the face leads the way.

- Breech—the baby's bottom is coming first  Breech presentations can be:
    - o Frank—baby's bottom is coming first, the legs are stretched up straight with the feet by the head
    - o Full (or Complete) - baby's legs are crossed Tailor-style
    - o Incomplete (footling, double footling or kneeling) - baby has one or both legs extended downward, either straight or bent at the knee.
- Transverse—the baby's shoulder is coming first.  A hand or arm may be extended into the birth canal. The baby cannot be born vaginally this way, it must be re-positioned to a longitudinal lie or be born by cesarean section.

# Baby's Station

Baby's "Station" refers to how far down the birth canal the presenting part has come.  "0" station is when the baby's presenting part is level with the ischial spines of the mother's bony pelvis.  When the baby is higher than the spines, the station may be "-1cm", "-2cm", "-3cm", etc. When the presenting part has passed the spines, the station is said to be "+1", "+2", "+3" centimeters below the spines.

# Tips for Optimal Positioning

Before 34 weeks, there is little concern about the baby's position unless it has been persistently in an unfavorable position (transverse, breech, posterior, etc.)  There are several exercises that you can do to help your baby get into the most favorable position for birth.

The most comfortable position for most mothers is when the baby is head-down, chin on its chest, and baby's back facing away from the mother's back.  These positions would be LOT, LOA, OA, ROA, and ROT.

Sometimes baby has a good reason to be in an "unfavorable" position and you will only know why after the baby is born.  Sometimes you will never know why.  Never force a baby to change positions. Gentle exercises that help baby get into a favorable position include crawling, "cat-back", "tail-wagging" and stair climbing. There are many more ideas for gently encouraging a baby to turn on www.SpinningBabies.com.

If the baby is transverse or breech, the above exercises are helpful, as are using a slant-board for inversion, homeopathics, acupuncture, and visualization; and using sound, warmth/cold, and vibration to encourage the baby to turn.

# 36 Week Home Visit

Most midwives will visit your home around 36 weeks, you will probably:
- Have a regular prenatal checkup and GBS swab
- Introduce all support people and discuss their roles
- Review instructions about when to contact your midwife and the quickest route to your home
- Discuss your preferences about Vitamin K, newborn screenings, Rhogam (if appropriate), Erythromycin, etc.
- Discuss your emergency back-up plan, including preferred routes and roles
- Check birth supplies and their location
- Discuss privacy - phone, email, social media, etc.
- Discuss postpartum plans - rest, home care, childcare for siblings, meals, placenta
- Discuss what to expect in labor
- Ask and answer questions

# Homebirth Checklist
- Hospital transfer/transport plan complete
- All birth supplies obtained and birth team knows their location
- Car ready for transport, if needed, and tank kept full of fuel
- Driver designated, in the case of transport
- Midwife and assistant phone numbers by the phone

# In Labor – What to Expect

Definitions:
- Antepartum - conception to onset of labor
- Intrapartum - onset of labor to completion of birth. The medical model defines the stages of labor as follows:
  - latent stage - 0 to 4 cm dilatation
  - first stage - 4 to 10 cm dilatation
  - second stage - full dilatation to birth of baby
  - third stage - baby birth to birth of placenta
  - fourth stage - first few hours following birth
- Postpartum - first few weeks following birth
- Dilation - the opening of the cervix
- Effacement - the thinning of the cervix

In reality stages of labor do not come in an orderly fashion, with one following obediently after another. Birth phases and stages overlap one another, starting and stopping, in a two-steps-forward, one-step-back fashion. The mother becomes pregnant, the baby grows, the uterus grows, the breasts grow, fat is stored for future use, hormones interplay. Gentle contractions hug the baby at irregular intervals, the contractions become stronger and more rhythmic then fade away. The cervix softens, preparing for its work. One day the mother notices that the contractions have become slowly stronger, interrupting what she is doing and demanding her attention. But when did this 'stage' begin? How do you mark the beginning of a continuum?

End of Pregnancy:
- Lightening - when baby drops down and engages in pelvis. First babies may drop a week or so before labor.

- Nesting urge - focused surge of energy to "get things ready"
- Weight loss, loose stools, dull low back ache, more pressure, need to pee often
- Baby may be less active
- Pre-labor (Braxton-Hicks) contractions may increase in frequency but remain irregular in strength and duration and rhythm. The more Braxton-Hicks, the shorter the labor.
- Practice labor (uterus warming up for its work) - this is not 'false' labor, it is effective at dilating and effacing the cervix.

Signs of Impending Labor:
- Regular contractions (80% begin this way) become longer, stronger and closer together. Labor will usually progress to birth within 16-24 hours for first birth and shorter with each subsequent labor. Though plan to be in this for the long haul.
- Blessed show - loss of healthy mucus seal... stretchy, egg-white consistency, may be pink or bloody tinged due to capillary breakage as cervix opens and pulls away from membranes... great or small amount which you may or may not notice. Usually labor begins in 24-48 hours after the loss of the mucous plug. Plan for 48 hours of labor, however, so you are not discouraged if your labor takes "only" 36 hours! Sometimes it takes a long time!
- Water breaking - usually happens when deep in labor but may be the first sign. Fluid should be clear and odorless.
- Pre-labor Rupture Of Membranes (PROM) - breaking without onset of contractions. This can be a normal variation of labor. If this happens, your midwife will check baby's heart tones and observe color of water. Heart tones should be in the normal range and water should be clear and without foul odor. Put nothing in the vagina: no sex, no baths, no fingers, etc. Increase fluids, echinacea, vitamin C, lemon, and garlic. If baby is not ready, the bag can reseal. Midwives handle PROM very differently than

hospitals.   Concerns for PROM include infection, baby's station, prolapsed cord, hand or other part; and loss of baby's protective bag and cushioning.

Patience:
- It is okay to do things that will encourage labor to start if baby is ready to be born.  These techniques will not cause labor to begin before baby is ready:
  o Walking
  o Curb-walking
  o Stair climbing
  o Gentle lovemaking
  o Gentle nipple stimulation
  o Female orgasm
  o Swallowing a capsule of Evening Primrose Oil morning and evening after 39 weeks of pregnancy is usually fine – ask your midwife
  o Drinking strong red raspberry leaf tea after 39 weeks is usually fine – ask your midwife
- Do NOT do anything to "induce" the labor, including suggestions that are all over the internet and other people think are "safe."  Inducing labor increases risks for both mother and baby.  Your best chance at a healthy, normal birth is to allow labor to begin and progress on its own!  Therefore, DO NOT:
  o Take castor oil: it can cause dehydration, hemorrhoids, meconium in the amniotic fluid, fetal distress, baby born before its ready to breathe, maternal high blood pressure and postpartum hemorrhage!
  o Use the herbs blue cohosh or black cohosh: they can cause too-strong of contractions, baby born before it's ready to breathe, fetal distress, and meconium in the water!
  o Take any drug or medicine to induce labor – DANGER!
    ▪ Pitocin – DANGER!
    ▪ Cytotec (Misoprostol) – DANGER!
  o Intentionally break the bag of water to induce labor – DANGER!

First Stage: the first stage of labor can be thought of

as having four phases: latent, active, transition and resting.

Latent phase
- Early labor, start-and-stop labor, or prodromal labor can go on for days or weeks before active labor begins.
- Cervical dilation, if you are checking, can be from 0 to 6 cm.
- This is usually the longest phase ranging form weeks to hours to moments. Practice sessions often happen during this phase.
- Contractions may feel mild to begin with and then increase in intensity and quantity.
- Some women describe them as crampy, gassy, or as a tightening. Some begin in the back and circle around to the lower abdomen, may begin low in front. They all will build, peak and gradually fade. Whatever her body does is normal for her.
- The mother may have periods of contractions and discomfort that fade away and return later.
- There is no set normal time for this phase.
- The mother should continue to eat well, rest and nap as much as possible, and do things to keep her mind off the contractions, trusting that her body knows exactly what to do.

Active phase
- Active labor usually lasts less than 24 hours.
- The cervix, if checked, will be dilated from 4 to 8 cm. This phase overlaps with the ones before and after. Its duration varies but is usually shorter than latent and marked by an obvious regularity of pattern. The mother can still chat between contractions. There may be more mucus and/or gush of blood as the cervix opens. As this phase progresses, she must focus on the feelings inside her body and pay attention to her labor. Each time she gets used to the contractions, they become more intense and she must focus to stay in tune with them.

- Mother should eat and drink throughout labor, especially as she gets to the end of this phase
- Mother should rest and nap as much as she can during labor
- BABY'S MOVEMENT: Baby should continue to move occasionally throughout labor. The mother should tell the midwife when she feels the baby move.
- The midwives will check the baby's heart rate regularly during labor. The heart rate should be in the normal range of 120-160 beats per minute (110-160 after the due date). If the range is outside of normal, the midwife may ask for a change of position or to get out of the birth tub for a while to see if the heart rate becomes normal again. It is normal for there to be a short dip in the heart rate during the pushing stage, as long as it comes quickly back to normal after each contraction.
- Help the mother to stay calm and breathe. The best way to do this is for you to stay calm and breathe.

Transition phase
- At the end of a normal First Stage, the contractions will be very close together and intense.
- The cervix, if checked, will be dilated from 7 to 10 cm.
- Some women feel hot/cold flashes, confused, irritable, shaky, and may vomit. This phase requires her full attention. Contractions may feel like they never quit, just as one is fading another is building. They may be every 2-3 minutes, lasting 1-2 minutes with double peaks.
- Most women will feel or say "I can't do this" at this time. The feelings of labor become overwhelming. The truth is that SHE IS DOING IT! It is normal to feel this way during transition.
- Encourage her to relax her bottom, relax her hips, relax her face, relax her jaw, relax her lips. Encourage her to open her eyes and look into yours. Breathe with her, slow and strong and deep.
- Counter-pressure on her back or bi-lateral hip pressure may feel good.

- A cool cloth on the forehead and warm compress across low abdomen are usually welcomed.
- Keep drinking and peeing. If baby is low, you may feel an urge to push.
- During this time the mother and her work become one thing - nothing else matters except birth. Beads of sweat may break out on her forehead. She will remove her clothing and her legs will naturally open. Breathing patterns will change, especially at the peak of each contraction.
- Pushing now may cause swelling of the cervix and impede descent of baby. Getting in the hands and knees position with counter back pressure usually helps. Breathing may need to become a rapid blow at peak of the contraction but return to deep, slow breathing as soon as urge passes. "Breathe for your baby."
- When urge becomes IRRESISTABLE, the mother may give a gentle push, just for a moment and at the very peak of the urge. If there is no pain with the push, or a good feeling, chances are she has entered the second stage.
- The midwife may check the cervix to make sure it is completely dilated before she begins pushing with every contraction.
- This is the time to urinate, get a drink and relax.

Diagram of Dilation and Effacement:

Cervix closed          1 cm dilated        2 cm dilated        3 cm dilated
not effaced            25% effaced         50% effaced         90% effaced

Resting Phase:
- Not all labors have a resting phase. But it is fine if yours does.
- The cervix, if checked, will not be measurable. It is open to its widest possibility and cannot be found when feeling around the sphere of the baby's head or bulging bag of water. We don't want to poke or puncture the bag. It is protecting the baby from the pressure of the contractions.
- The mother may become tired and need to eat and rest a bit when first stage ends and before second stage begins.

Second Stage (Pushing):
- This stage begins when the cervix is fully open to the same diameter as the baby's head (called "10 centimeters") and ends with the birth of the baby. This stage may take 1-2 hours for first time mothers and is usually shorter with each subsequent birth.
- As baby moves down, the lower back may ache and pressure on rectum causes an intense urge to push. If waters haven't broken, they usually will now.
- Encourage the mother to choose different positions.
- It is difficult to push a baby out with tightness in your bottom, thighs, throat, or forehead. Drop your chin, shoulders, mouth, knees, and bottom. Let the baby down and out. Squatting or sitting on a stool uses gravity and opens the pelvis. All effort for mother and baby is to get comfortable. Use stairs to shake down a baby that is acynclitic.
- Warm compresses and gentle perineal massage may feel good to the mother. Some women naturally reach down and touch or massage wherever they feel discomfort.
- The mother's movement and sounds will be exaggerated and deep. She will naturally make low grunting and growling "mama bear" sounds.
- She should get in whatever position she is most comfortable (or least uncomfortable!) All positions have advantages - standing, squatting, left side lying, semi-sitting, hands and knees.

- The mother will begin to feel the urge to push, as if she has to poop. She may even say she needs to go to the toilet, thinking she needs to have a bowel movement. If so, someone should go with her, so she won't push the baby into the toilet.
- Pushing should be done at the peak of a contraction and only when the mother has the irresistible urge to push. Throughout the rest of the contraction, she should be breathing.
- The mother should have a sip of juice or bite of banana in between pushes. This will give her and the baby energy to finish the birth.
- Breathe deeply and slowly between the pushes. This will provide oxygen to her uterus so it can push effectively and provide oxygen to the baby so it will be in good condition at birth.
- Encourage her with phrases like:
  - "You're doing it."
  - "You're doing great."
  - "Breathe for your baby."
  - "Baby's coming."
  - "You never have to do that contraction again."
- During the pushing phase, a dip in the heart rate may be heard as the baby's head descends through the birth canal. This is normal *if* it is only for a brief few seconds at the peak of a contraction, does not dip lower than 100 beats per minute or so, and comes back up to baseline immediately following the contraction.
- The mother's perineum will begin to bulge outward when she pushes. This means the baby's head is coming down. She may poop a little during these pushes.
- A little of the baby's head or bag of water will become visible as the labia presses open during a push. Then it will go back inside between pushes. This is normal. With each push more and more of the baby's head or bag of water will be visible.
- When the head is visible, the midwife or support person should tell the mother "I see the baby." She may want to look with a mirror to see it for herself.

- The mother may feel her vagina and perineum stretching and burning in what has been called "the ring of fire." Help her relax and breathe and resist pushing to prevent tearing.
- As the head emerges, it should be a pale pink or pale lavender color, usually very wrinkled and may or may not have much hair. Overlapping suture lines may be prominent and may be mistaken for a cord over the head.
- When the head is half-way out and does not go back in between the contractions, the head is "crowning". Have the mom pant if she has to in order not to push. Let her body slowly push the rest of the head out without her adding to the body's own efforts.
- Encourage the mother to touch her baby's head. Often, if the mother keeps her hand on the baby's head, she will find it easier to push the baby out gently instead of too-fast.
- The forehead will slowly be born, followed by the eyes, nose, mouth and chin!
- If there is a cord around the neck (incidence: 30%) the midwife will loop it over the head, or hold the baby near the mother as she pushes out the body, then unwrap the cord.
- If there is no cord around the neck, the mother may push with the next contraction.
- The head will slowly rotate before the shoulders are born.
- If the shoulders get stuck (shoulder dystocia, incidence: 1%), the midwife will direct the mother to change positions, which usually frees the shoulder. Rarely, the midwife will have to maneuver the shoulders and help the baby out.
- The shoulders will emerge, followed by the body and legs.

Third Stage (birth of baby to birth of placenta):
- The birth is not complete until the placenta is born and baby and mother are both stable. This is time to focus on baby and fall in love, while waiting for the placenta. This is not the time to begin calling family and friends. You do not want to divert attention

from the mother at this point, and you definitely do not want people showing up at the house before the placenta is born and everyone is cleaned up and ready to meet the extended family!

- The baby should be placed immediately on the mother's bare chest, so baby will be warmed and comforted by skin-to-skin contact with mother.
- The midwife will monitor the baby and mother. Most babies are not breathing at the moment of birth. It may take 30 to 45 seconds before they do, which seems like an eternity! If the baby needs help breathing, the midwife will not hesitate to help.
- The baby does not have to cry in order to breathe. Some babies cry with their first breaths, others simply begin breathing as they look around at their new world.
- There is no hurry to cut the cord. It can be cut hours or days later, or not at all. If or when the cord is cut, it MUST be done with sterile clamp or string and sterile scissors.
- The baby's suckling reflex is strongest in the first hour of life. If this precious opportunity is lost by busy-ness (like weighing and measuring the baby) it may be much harder to get the baby latched on later. Therefore, the baby should be kept skin-to-skin with the mother so he or she can latch on when the urge is strongest. The baby will be alert and may give cues s/he is ready to nurse:
  o Baby turns its head toward the breast
  o Smells and licks the breast and nipple
  o Opens its mouth
- Keep the baby near the nipple so he or she can latch on whenever he or she is ready. Do not separate the baby from the mother.
- There is usually no hurry to deliver the placenta. It usually takes 15 to 45 minutes for before you see signs that the placenta is ready to be born. The midwife will gently assist the placenta delivery. Signs the placenta is ready:
  o Contractions/cramps resume: the mother may complain that she feels crampy. These are

uterine contractions preparing to push out the placenta.
- o Placenta "show": there is bleeding when the placenta has released from the uterine wall and is ready to be born. Normal blood loss with the placenta is two cups or less.
- o Cord lengthening: you may notice the cord comes out an inch or two farther when the placenta begins to come down.
- Safe and natural ways to encourage the placenta to come:
  - o Nurse the baby
  - o Have the mother sit upright.
  - o Empty the bladder – have the mother go pee
  - o If she is strong and not dizzy or too tired, she can squat over a pad or bowl to birth the placenta.
- The placenta looks dark red and meaty. The midwife will put it in a bowl or on a pad, and examine it to make sure it is intact and normal.
- Mother's bleeding should be minimal. It is normal to have a gush of dark blood when changing positions, especially when standing up after laying down for a while. It should not be a constant flow.
- The midwife will cut the cord, or assist as you cut the cord, around the time of the newborn exam. You want to wait until the cord has stopped pulsing at the baby's belly-button before cutting. This usually takes about an hour.
- The midwife will examine the mother for tears and make repairs if needed. The mother will need stitches only about 20% of the time. If there is a very bad tear, it may be necessary to go to a hospital to have it repaired, but most small tears can be sutured at home.
  - o If there is any skid mark or tearing, with or without stitches, the mother should be advised to:
    - ▪ keep her knees together for two weeks, avoiding stairs

- increase vitamin C and garlic intake to ward of infection
- use a peri-bottle to spray her vagina and perineum when using the toilet, letting her pad catch any drips instead of wiping with toilet paper. Particles of toilet paper stick to the wound and can cause an infection. Use baby wipes to gently clean after a bowel movement.
- take two healing herbal stiz baths per day

- Congratulations! The birth is complete! Get a drink and some food for the mother and yourself. Enjoy your baby! Now is the time to share your joy with family and friends!

Fourth Stage: Baby Moon (the first few weeks postpartum)

- The first few days are critical for laying the foundation of health and happiness between mother and your baby. Mother should stay in bed with baby nursing for the first three days. The two should never be separated except to bathe or use the toilet. Food should be brought in to her and visitors kept to a few family members or special friends.
- Mother should stay in her pajamas for the first week. Pajamas signal to visitors that she is resting—not entertaining. Give all visitors a task. Grandmother starting the laundry and best friend washing the dishes will be a great help.
- Expect a heavy discharge for the first 12-24 hours. There may be a few clots and pads should be changed frequently. Mother should nurse the baby often and urinate at least every two hours while awake to decrease blood loss. Check the uterus periodically during the first 12 hours. It should feel hard and the size of a grapefruit. If it is not, massage the uterus or get the baby to nurse.
  - Bleeding should not soak 2 pads within ½ hour. If it does, call your midwife.
  - After the first 24-48 hours, bleeding should be like a normal period, decreasing in flow and getting lighter or brownish in color.

- o If it should come back bright red, then activity has probably been excessive. REST!
  - o The flow should not have any bad odor, it should smell like your period. A foul odor is a sign of infection. Please call your midwife if it smells bad.
- Mother should stay off her feet the first week, getting up only to go to the bathroom and to shower/bathe. Have her meals brought to her.
- Gradually add light activity the second week, resting when tired and napping daily with baby. Arrange for someone else to help with other children, meals and housework. Do not lift anything heavier than baby for the first few weeks. Being too active can result in increased bleeding, feeling blue and reduced milk production now, and prolapsed organs later in life.
- If baby shows any signs of jaundice (yellow skin) within the first 24 hours, call your midwife.
- Nurse your baby often, at least every 2 hours. Anytime the baby cries, offer the breast. Make sure the baby is positioned tummy to tummy and is taking in as much of the areola, the brown area surrounding the nipple, as possible.
  - o For the first few days, if baby doesn't wake up to nurse after two hours, wake him or her up. It is important to set good habits early and create a sufficient milk supply.
  - o After the initial 3 weeks, you can start to follow baby's feeding patterns. Remember that it takes a full month or more for you both to learn to breastfeed. You will have both good and bad days. The important thing to acknowledge is that baby's body knows when the supply needs to be increased and will let you know by nursing more frequently. You may have days when you do nothing but nurse. Listen to baby and don't offer anything else and the supply will adjust to be perfect. (Sucking is as important as food is to a baby.)
  - o Baby should have nothing but breast milk for at least 6 months.

- o Breastfed babies require no water.
- o Avoid the bottle unless separation is necessary, and then only after the initial supply is established, 1 month minimum.
- o Pacifiers interfere with nursing and should not be used.
- o Transition to new parenthood will be easier if baby is allowed to sleep with mother.
- Drink plenty of water.
- Continue eating well and taking your vitamins. Mother should not be in such a hurry to lose weight that she deprives herself and baby of protein and calories.
- The umbilical cord stump dries up from lack of blood supply, not from lack of water. Therefore baby may be bathed.
- Do not use soaps or other cleaning products on baby's cord. Keep the cord dry and above the diaper line. Don't put anything on it. You may sponge bathe baby with water or oil avoiding the cord area. The cord has a normal smell like drying meat. It should not smell foul like rotting flesh or have any puss oozing from it. The skin around the belly button should not be red or inflamed. If it is, contact your midwife.
- You should wait until 2-3 weeks after all bloody vaginal discharge has stopped before having sex. For those who wish to use birth control, it should be considered immediately. Natural Family Planning works very well when done correctly. Diaphragms and condoms are relatively safe. Hormonal forms of birth control, like the pill, shot, implants, and cervical ring may cause future problems ranging from hormonal imbalances to cancer, and should never be used while nursing.
- Enjoy your baby and give him/her plenty of skin to skin contact with both mom and dad. It is impossible to spoil a newborn baby. Don't be afraid to meet all her needs immediately. It will give him or her the security he or she needs and he or she will be a much easier baby.

# *Waterbirth*

The use of water during labor eases the pain of labor. Hot water showering on the back; warm, wet compresses on the perineum; and even submersion in a tub of warm water have all been used to help the mom relax. Imagine the spinal cord as a network of couriers carrying messages from the body up to the brain. In theory, messages about sensations closer to the top of the spine take precedence over messages coming from farther away from the brain. Therefore, a message about how painful a labor contraction feels will be partially blocked by a message about how good warm water higher on the back feels.

If you want to try submersion in water as a pain-relief technique, I recommend waiting until the pain has built to a level where it is hard to cope using other techniques (distraction, relaxation, breathing, back rub, counter-pressure). You will get much more benefit from the water if you don't get in too soon, and getting in way too early can stop your labor!

A baby is stimulated to take its first breath when air touches the face. If the baby is born underwater, air does not touch the face at the moment of birth, so the baby does not attempt to breathe. Even if it did, it would not be able to because the alveoli of the lungs are filled with fluid. You can't add more water to a cup that is already full. When the baby is born, it is immediately brought to the surface and up onto mother's chest, face down so any water in the mouth will run out. Air touches the face and baby is stimulated to breathe. The first breaths, whether baby was born in water or not, force the fluid in the alveoli through the thin membrane of the alveoli walls and into the tissue of the lungs and the baby begins to breathe. The baby does not cough our spit out this fluid, as is sometimes taught.

When a waterbirth is planned, or even just a water-labor, there should always be a "landing pad" (a foam

mat, sleeping bag, or several thick blankets) nearby
that can be used to make a quick bed in case the
mother needs or wants to get out at the last minute.

# Adrenaline

Fear affects labor and birth. In the animal kingdom, a mare,
ewe, cow, or doe will stop laboring if a predator comes near.
She will close down and hold back her offspring until she is
in a safe location. The same is true of women. Though
doctors and hospital staff will disagree, a woman's cervix
can actually close down to a smaller dilation than it was an
hour before.

Adrenaline is a hormone that is excreted whenever a woman
feels unsafe, like in an unfamiliar location, around strangers
or someone she does not trust. Adrenaline inhibits cervical
dilation, and can reverse it. Ina May Gaskin, the famous
midwife from Tennessee, attributes this reversal of dilation
to what she calls "the sphincter law." Sphincters are ring-
shaped muscles that surround the opening to various
organs like the stomach, bladder and anus. Sphincters open
better in privacy, and warm, familiar, comfortable places.
Imagine how hard it would be to have a bowel movement on
a toilet right out in the open in the middle of a busy
shopping mall, with strangers bustling around you. Now
imagine how hard it would be to give birth in a busy
hospital suite, with strangers bustling around, poking you
with needles, sticking their hands inside your vagina
without even introducing themselves or asking permission.
The cervix is not an actual sphincter, but it behaves in the
same way.

# Fear

Before and during labor, a mother may be fearful and
unable to trust her body. This can affect the labor pattern
and birth outcome, whether or not the thing she feared
actually came to be.

Some people feel strongly that you should never talk about
your fears or they may come true. I believe if you have a

fear, the fear already exists! Talking about it cannot make it more real, but can help the person to determine if the fear is likely to happen or a rare occurrence; deal with the fear and help the person to have a plan in mind what she or he would do if the fearful thing came to be.

What is a possible fear that a mother, father, family member or midwife may have? Is this likely to happen? What plan could be made to deal with this if it happened? Is the fear real? Is it an intuition that something is wrong? Or is it just a fear that is standing in the way, hindering the mother from fully relaxing into her labor-work?

## *Prayers and Affirmations*

Positive prayers and affirmations can be used when your fear is growing and you have an inner sense that everything is fine, the fear is not real. If it is just an untrue fear, a positive prayer or affirmation may be just the thing to get you past it.

By "positive" I mean that we do not pray about or think of the thing we do not want. Instead, we pray for and think about the thing that we do want!

For example, when I pray for a birth, I never think "the baby does not get stuck" or "there will not be very much bleeding" or "the mother will not tear." Instead I pray that "the baby descends and is born easily," "the placenta is born whole and compete and the uterus contracts hard like it is supposed to," and "the perineum and vagina are intact." See the difference? Do not try to pray away what you do not want. Visualize what you do want to happen. Imagine yourself relaxing every muscle in your body. Imagine your baby emerging, head first, from your body. The baby is pink and strong and nurses right away. The milk flows freely. The placenta is born and the uterus contracts as normal. The family falls in love with each other and bonds right away. Ask and you shall receive!

# When Giving Birth is Difficult

Sometimes birth is not what we expected and leaves the mother with a feeling of loss. Loss can take many different forms, from mild to severe. Loss can mean the death of a baby, but it is more frequently a milder form of loss. Loss of the perfect birth ideal, a long hard labor when you were expecting it to be easy, loss of control of your body, loss of emotional state, emergence of physical sensations that remind you of past sexual trauma, loss of bowel control during pushing, birth via cesarean surgery when you wanted a vaginal birth, loss of control over your day-to-day and how you choose to spend it, postpartum health challenges. Change. Life. Unpredictability.

Sometimes the outcome of the birth is unexpected. An unexpected loss will hit the family harder than a loss that was expected. Do not listen to people who try to minimize your feelings or experience. It is appropriate to feel the pain of sadness after a loss. No one can feel it for you. Avoiding your feelings or "stuffing it down" will wreck your health and the feelings will re-surface later—probably at the least convenient of times. Feel your sadness now, go through the grief cycle. You will come out on the other side and be whole again. Talk to someone you trust about your feelings, someone who will listen and not try to tell you what you should be thinking.

# Postpartum Instructions

Mother
- Expect heavy discharge the first 12-24 hours. You may pass clots and will need to change pads frequently. Never use tampons or a Diva cup during postpartum flow. Nurse baby often and urinate at least every two hours while awake to decrease blood loss. Check the uterus periodically during the first 12 hours. It should feel hard and the size of a grapefruit. If it is not, massage it and get the baby to

nurse.
- Bleeding should not soak a maxi-pad within ½ hour. If it does, call immediately. After the first 24 hours, bleeding should be like a normal period, decreasing in flow and getting lighter or brownish in color. If it should come back bright red, then activity has probably been excessive. Rest!
- Flow should not have bad odor, it should smell like your period. Please call if it smells bad or the color does not look right.
- Your uterus should feel hard, round, grapefruit-sized, and be below your navel. If it's not firm, massage it and get baby nursing. Keeping your bladder empty will help keep your uterus normal.
- You should have a normal body temperature. If your temperature is over 100.4° after drinking lots of fluids, call your midwife.
- Your pulse should be normal. If you feel your pulse is racing, you can count how many beats per minute. It should be less than 100 beats per minute. If it's more than that, with heavy bleeding, call your midwife immediately.
- You should pee and poop normally. Spray your vulva using your peri bottle when you pee if you have any stinging. Eat lots of raw fruit and veggies, drink lots of water, and avoid constipating foods like meats and cheese until you have passed your first bowel movement. Do not strain on the toilet. Put your feet on a footstool to keep your knees higher than your hips. Do not "push" the bowel movement. Let it slide out on its own.
- Stay off your feet the first week, get up only to go to the bathroom and to shower/bathe. Have your meals brought to you. Gradually add light activity the second week, resting when tired and napping daily with baby. Arrange for someone to help with children, meals and housework. Do not lift anything heavier than baby for the first few weeks. Doing too much results in increased bleeding, feeling blue and reduced milk production.
- Sometime between day 7 through day 10, the uterus

involution causes the site of placental attachment to slough off. This causes a temporary increase in flow. If you go out, be prepared with a maxi pad in your diaper bag!

- You will have an easier transition if baby sleeps with you.
- Continue eating well and taking your vitamins. Don't be in such a rush to lose weight that you and baby are deprived of protein and calories.
- Drink plenty of water. Drink every time your baby nurses.
- You should wait until 2-3 weeks after all discharge has stopped before having sex. For those who wish to use birth control, it should be used immediately. Natural Family Planning works very well when done correctly and has no harmful side effects. Diaphragms and condoms are relatively safe. Hormonal forms of birth control (like the pill, shot, implant, nuva ring, IUDs, etc.) may cause future problems like hormonal imbalances and cancer, and should not be used while breastfeeding.
- Call your midwife if you have any abnormal signs, such as fainting, severe headache, severe pain in the abdomen, legs or chest, spots before the eyes, despair, great anxiety or inability to cope.

## Baby

- Baby should pee and poop within 24 hours. After that, baby should give you 8 to 12 wet and/or dirty diapers every 24 hours. If less than that, baby needs to nurse more frequently. The first few days, baby's bowel movements are very tarry and black. This is called meconium. It is made mostly of old red blood cells that have been processed by the liver and are ready to be eliminated. Oil the baby's bottom when diapering to avoid having to scrape the meconium from the skin! The more baby nurses, the more quickly this tarry stool will be eliminated, and the less jaundice the baby will have. The bowel movement should be the color and consistency of yellow mustard within a few days.

- Baby's skin, lips and tongue should be pink. If baby has yellow skin within the first 24 hours, call your midwife.
- Baby's temperature, taken under the arm with a thermometer, will be between 96 and 98 degrees. If it's less than 96 or over 98, adjust the room temperature, put baby skin-to-skin with mom and cover with a blanket (if temp was low) or unbundled (if temp was warm). Call midwife if the temperature does not normalize.
- Baby's breathing should not be labored. Baby should not be grunting or flaring her nostrils. The skin should not retract under the ribs with the breath. Normal respirations per minute are between 30 and 60 breaths per minute. Call your midwife if you are concerned.
- Nurse baby often, at least every 2 hours. Anytime baby cries, offer the breast. Make sure baby is tummy-to-tummy with mama and baby's mouth is centered on areola (brown area around nipple) and taking in as much of the nipple as possible.
- If baby doesn't wake to nurse after two hours, wake her up. This is important to build a sufficient milk supply. After 3 weeks, you can start to follow baby's patterns. It takes a month or more for you both to learn to breastfeed. You will have good and bad days. When the supply needs to increase, baby will naturally nurse more frequently. Some days you may do nothing but nurse. Listen to baby, don't offer supplements or pacifiers and the supply will be perfect.
- Breastfed babies require no water after the milk comes in. A sunken front "soft spot" indicates dehydration. Baby needs only breast milk for at least 6 months.
- Avoid using a bottle unless separation is necessary, and then only after the initial supply is established, 1 month minimum. Sucking is as important as food to a baby.
- Pacifiers interfere with nursing and should not be used.

- Keep the cord dry and above the diaper line. Don't put anything on it. You may sponge bathe baby with water or oil avoiding the cord area. You may also take baby in the bath with you. Wetting the cord in the bath will not harm it. The area around the cord should not be red or hot. The cord has an odor, but not a foul odor. If the cord smells like something rotten, call your midwife.
- Give baby lots of skin-to-skin contact with mom and dad.
- It is impossible to spoil a newborn baby. Don't be afraid to meet all her needs immediately. It will give her the security she needs and she will be a much easier baby.
- Please call your midwife with any questions or concerns, including excessive sleepiness/hard to wake (wake baby to feed every 2-3 hours), hyperirritability or extreme reaction to ordinary stimulation like diaper changing, picking baby up, etc., jaundice (yellow skin) on the first day, poor feeding, not at all interested in feeding, or exhausted by it.

## How to Make More Milk

These are general rules for increasing milk production. Remember that there will be about 24 hours between the time you start programming your body to make more milk and the time it comes in.

- **Slow down!** Slow the pace of your life. Do less. Take your time.
- **Nurse!** Increase the number of feeding sessions. Frequency of feedings provides more effective stimulation for increased production than does the length of each session. Private feeding sessions are preferable to those in a busy, distracting atmosphere.
- **Eat well!** Eat wholesome foods and cut out junk foods and empty calories.
- **Drink!** Drink plenty of pure water. Always drink when baby nurses. Borage tea and red raspberry leaf tea may help to boost milk production.

- **Sleep!** Get plenty of sleep. Sleep when your baby sleeps. Do not use baby's naptime as a chance to catch up on housework.
- **Enjoy!** Be sure to kiss and cuddle and play with your baby during these sessions. If she gets frustrated, take a 5 to 10 minute play break and then put her back to the breast.

"It should be comforting to know that with the right diet and the right lifestyle and atmosphere, nearly every woman who wants to breastfeed her baby will be able to do so. Biologically, this is true."          - Ina May Gaskin

# *Placenta*

As a Native American Medicine Woman and Midwife, I was trained to use the placenta for its intended purposes as a food and a medicine. I consider it part of God's birth kit!

What was a taboo subject for me to speak of a few years ago has blossomed into a topic that everyone wants to talk about! A sliver of raw placenta under the tongue or chewed and swallowed will stop a hemorrhage. It can be used to decrease postpartum bleeding, prevent and treat "baby blues" and postpartum depression, bring emotional balance, increase milk supply, save for later to treat premenstrual syndrome and all kinds of menstrual problems and pre-menopausal and menopausal problems. In China, women save their placenta capsules to use during the hormonal changes of menopause.

Your placenta grew inside of you, producing hormones by you and for you. The hormones contained in your placenta were not manufactured in some laboratory. They are perfect for your body. But it gets even better: the placenta contains every known enzyme. How, I cannot tell you, but ongoing research about the power of the placenta is mind-boggling!

Instructions for drying and encapsulating your own placenta, can be found online or from your midwife. Your midwife may also have a referral to someone who will do it for you.

## Birth Story

Your birth story is important. Take time now, while it's fresh in your mind, to get the details on paper. The experience starts to fade all too soon. When you are ready, you can share your story with your child or with other women who need to know that they, too, can do it.

# About the Author

Deborah Duren-Smithey is a wife, mother, grandmother, and Certified Professional Midwife. Her three children and one grandchild were all born at home. She has a homebirth practice and attends births in southwest Missouri.